GALLBLADDER DIET MASTERY

Regain Control of Your Health

Adams .U. Morris

TABLE OF CONTENTS

CHAPTER 1

Introduction - Understanding the Gallbladder and the Importance of a Gallbladder Diet

In this opening chapter, we embark on a journey to understand the often-overlooked organ in our body: the gallbladder. It may seem like a small, insignificant pouch nestled beneath our liver, but it plays a crucial role in our digestive system. Our gallbladder's health is something we seldom think about until it starts causing problems. In this chapter, we'll explore what the gallbladder does, why it's so vital, and why adopting a gallbladder-friendly diet can be a game-changer for your overall well-being.

The Gallbladder Unveiled

Imagine your digestive system as a well-choreographed dance, with each organ playing a unique role. The gallbladder, a pear-shaped organ, is the "stage manager" of this performance. Its primary job is to store and concentrate bile, a yellow-green fluid produced by the liver. Bile is like nature's detergent; it breaks down fats in the foods we eat, making them easier to digest.

The gallbladder releases bile into the small intestine, especially when we consume fatty meals. This burst of bile helps emulsify fats, turning them into tiny droplets that digestive enzymes can more effectively process. Without a functioning gallbladder, this process becomes erratic, leading to discomfort and poor digestion.

Why the Gallbladder Matters

You might be wondering, "If it's so small, can't we live without it?" Well, the gallbladder may not be vital for survival, but it certainly plays a pivotal role in our daily lives. Here are a few reasons why it's essential:

1. **Fat Digestion**: As mentioned earlier, the gallbladder's main job is to aid in fat digestion. Fats are essential nutrients, and without proper digestion, you may not absorb the fat-soluble vitamins A, D, E, and K as efficiently.

2. **Digestive Comfort**: A well-functioning gallbladder contributes to smooth digestion. When it's not working correctly, you might experience symptoms like bloating, gas, and diarrhea, particularly after meals rich in fats.

3. **Gallstones**: One of the most common gallbladder issues is the formation of gallstones. These are hard deposits that can block the flow of bile, causing intense pain and even requiring surgical removal of the gallbladder.

4. **Digestive Disorders**: Problems with the gallbladder can contribute to or exacerbate other digestive disorders, such as irritable bowel syndrome (IBS) and acid reflux.

Now that we've highlighted why the gallbladder is crucial, let's delve into why a specialized diet is essential when you're dealing with gallbladder issues.

The Need for a Gallbladder Diet

To keep your gallbladder happy and your digestive system in

harmony, a gallbladder diet can be a lifesaver. But why is it necessary? Let's explore a few key reasons:

1. **Minimizing Gallstone Formation**: If you've ever had a gallstone or are at risk of developing one, dietary choices play a pivotal role in preventing their formation. A gallbladder-friendly diet can help control the factors that contribute to stone development, such as excessive cholesterol and inadequate gallbladder contractions.

2. **Symptom Management**: Individuals with gallbladder issues often experience unpleasant symptoms like pain, nausea, and digestive upset. A diet tailored to support gallbladder health can minimize these symptoms, enhancing your overall quality of life.

3. **Preserving Gallbladder Function**: In some cases, gallbladder problems can lead to inflammation (cholecystitis) or impaired gallbladder function. By adopting a gallbladder diet, you can reduce stress on the

gallbladder and potentially prevent the need for surgical removal.

4. **Enhancing Digestion**: A well-balanced gallbladder diet isn't just about avoiding certain foods; it's also about including those that promote efficient digestion. This can lead to less discomfort, better nutrient absorption, and improved overall well-being.

Now that we've established why a gallbladder diet is essential, you might be wondering what exactly it entails. In the subsequent chapters of this book, we'll explore the specifics of a gallbladder-friendly diet, including the foods to avoid, those to embrace, and practical meal planning tips.

But before we dive into those details, it's crucial to recognize that a gallbladder diet isn't one-size-fits-all. Just like our bodies, our gallbladders are unique. Some people can tolerate certain foods better than others, and individual sensitivities may vary. Therefore, this book aims to provide you with a comprehensive understanding of gallbladder health and dietary guidelines. It's important to consult with a healthcare professional or a registered dietitian to create a personalized gallbladder diet plan that suits your specific needs.

In the subsequent chapters, we will explore various aspects of a gallbladder diet, including the foods you should avoid to prevent aggravating gallbladder issues, the importance of maintaining a balanced diet rich in lean proteins, healthy fats, and fiber, and practical tips for meal planning, portion control, and lifestyle factors that can influence gallbladder health. We'll also provide you with a selection of gallbladder-friendly recipes and sample meal plans to help you get started on your journey to better digestive health.

In closing, your gallbladder is a small but mighty organ that deserves your attention and care. By understanding its role in digestion and adopting a gallbladder-friendly diet, you can take significant steps toward improving your digestive comfort and overall well-being. So, let's embark on this journey together, exploring the fascinating world of

gallbladder health and the power
of nutrition in supporting it.

CHAPTER 2

Understanding Gallbladder Problems

In this chapter, we delve into the world of gallbladder problems. These can be painful, frustrating, and significantly impact your quality of life. By gaining a deeper understanding of common gallbladder conditions, their symptoms, and risk factors, you'll be better equipped to navigate the challenges they pose and make informed decisions about your health.

Gallbladder Problems Unveiled

The gallbladder, as we learned in the previous chapter, is a small yet crucial organ in our digestive system. It's designed to store and concentrate bile, which is essential for breaking down fats in the foods we eat. However, like any part of our body, the gallbladder can face issues. Here are some common gallbladder problems:

1. **Gallstones (Cholelithiasis):**
   - **What Are They?**: Gallstones are small, hard deposits that

form in the gallbladder. They can be made of cholesterol or bilirubin, a component of bile.

- ○ **Symptoms**:
  Gallstones can cause intense pain, often referred to as a "gallbladder attack." This pain typically occurs in the upper-right abdomen and may radiate to the back or shoulder blades. Other symptoms include nausea and vomiting.

- **Risk Factors**: Gallstones are more common in individuals who are overweight, women, over the age of 40, or have a family history of gallstones. Rapid weight loss and pregnancy can also increase the risk.

2. **Cholecystitis (Inflammation of the Gallbladder)**:

   - **What Is It?**: Cholecystitis is an inflammation of the gallbladder, often caused by gallstones blocking the bile ducts. It can be acute (sudden and severe) or chronic (long-term).

- **Symptoms**: Acute cholecystitis presents with severe abdominal pain, fever, and sometimes jaundice (yellowing of the skin and eyes). Chronic cholecystitis may lead to recurring, milder pain after meals.
- **Risk Factors**: Gallstones are the primary risk factor for cholecystitis. Obesity

and a high-fat diet can increase the likelihood of developing gallstones.

3. **Biliary Dyskinesia**:

   - **What Is It?**: Biliary dyskinesia is a disorder in which the gallbladder doesn't contract as it should, leading to impaired bile flow. It can cause symptoms similar to gallstones.

   - **Symptoms**: Individuals with biliary dyskinesia often experience abdominal pain, bloating, and indigestion, especially after eating fatty foods.

- **Risk Factors**: The exact cause of biliary dyskinesia isn't always clear, but it can be associated with previous gallbladder surgery or inflammation.

4. **Gallbladder Polyps**:

- **What Are They?**: Gallbladder polyps are growths that develop on the gallbladder wall. They are usually noncancerous but can, in some cases, become malignant.

- **Symptoms**: Polyps typically don't cause symptoms on their own. They are usually discovered incidentally during imaging tests for other conditions.

- **Risk Factors**: Risk factors for gallbladder polyps include age, obesity, and certain chronic conditions.

5. **Choledocholithiasis (Bile Duct Stones)**:

- **What Is It?**: These are gallstones that

move from the gallbladder into the common bile duct, which carries bile from the liver and gallbladder to the small intestine.

- ○ **Symptoms**: Choledocholithiasis can cause abdominal pain, jaundice, and pancreatitis (inflammation of the pancreas).
- ○ **Risk Factors**: The risk is higher for individuals with a history of gallstones or

certain medical conditions affecting the bile ducts.

Now that we have a grasp of these common gallbladder issues, let's move on to understanding their symptoms.

Spotting Gallbladder Problem Symptoms

Gallbladder problems often share common symptoms, but the severity and duration can vary. It's essential to recognize these signs and seek medical attention if you suspect an issue. Here are some common symptoms:

1. **Abdominal Pain**: Pain or discomfort in the upper-right abdomen is a hallmark symptom. It may be sharp and intense, often occurring after meals, particularly those high in fats.

2. **Nausea and Vomiting**: Gallbladder problems can lead to nausea and vomiting, especially during or after meals.

3. **Bloating and Gas**: Some individuals experience bloating and excessive gas, which can be quite uncomfortable.

4. **Indigestion**: Digestive disturbances, including indigestion and heartburn, can be symptoms of gallbladder problems.

5. **Changes in Stool**: Gallbladder issues may lead to changes in stool color, often making it lighter in color than usual.

6. **Jaundice**: Yellowing of the skin and eyes (jaundice) can occur if gallstones block the bile ducts, preventing the flow of bile.

7. **Fever and Chills**: In cases of acute cholecystitis, fever

and chills may accompany severe abdominal pain.

Understanding these symptoms can help you identify potential gallbladder problems early, allowing for prompt medical evaluation and treatment. If you or someone you know experiences these symptoms, it's crucial to consult a healthcare professional.

Assessing Risk Factors

While anyone can develop gallbladder problems, certain factors can increase your risk. Being aware of these risk factors can help you take preventive measures. Here are some key risk factors for gallbladder problems:

1. **Age**: Gallstones become more common as people age, particularly after the age of 40.
2. **Gender**: Women are more likely than men to develop gallstones, partly due to hormonal changes, including pregnancy and the use of birth control pills.
3. **Obesity**: Excess body weight, especially around the waist, is a significant risk factor for gallstones and related conditions.

4. **Family History**: If your family has a history of gallstones, your risk may be higher.

5. **Rapid Weight Loss**: Losing weight too quickly can increase the risk of gallstones. Gradual, steady weight loss is recommended.

6. **Dietary Choices**: Diets high in unhealthy fats and low in fiber can contribute to gallstone formation.

7. **Certain Medical Conditions**: Conditions such as diabetes, liver disease, and Crohn's disease

can increase the risk of gallbladder problems.

8. **Medications**: Some medications, like cholesterol-lowering drugs, can contribute to gallstone formation.

By recognizing these risk factors, you can make lifestyle adjustments to reduce your chances of developing gallbladder issues. For example, maintaining a healthy weight through diet and exercise, avoiding rapid weight loss diets, and making dietary choices that promote gallbladder health can all be beneficial.

In conclusion, this chapter has shed light on the various gallbladder problems that individuals can face, their symptoms, and the risk factors associated with them. Having a solid understanding of these aspects is the first step towards proactively managing your gallbladder health. In the following chapters, we'll delve into the practical aspects of maintaining a gallbladder-friendly diet, including foods to avoid, foods to embrace, meal planning, and lifestyle factors that can influence gallbladder health. Armed with this knowledge, you'll

be better prepared to take control
of your digestive well-being.

CHAPTER 3

Gallbladder Diet Basics

Welcome to Chapter 3 of our exploration into the world of gallbladder health and dietary choices. In this chapter, we'll dive deep into the fundamental principles of a gallbladder diet. You'll discover why dietary adjustments are crucial for supporting gallbladder health, the role of fats in gallbladder function, and the importance of incorporating low-fat and high-fiber foods into your daily meals.

Why a Special Diet for the Gallbladder?

You might wonder why you need to modify your diet to cater to your gallbladder. After all, isn't it just one organ in a complex digestive system? The truth is, what you eat significantly influences your gallbladder's health and your overall digestive comfort.

1. **Managing Gallstones**: If you've ever experienced the excruciating pain of gallstones, you know how important it is to avoid triggering another attack. Certain dietary choices can

help minimize the risk of gallstone formation and reduce the likelihood of future episodes.

2. **Preventing Gallbladder Inflammation**: Gallstones can lead to cholecystitis, the inflammation of the gallbladder. By adopting a gallbladder-friendly diet, you can reduce the chances of gallstone-related complications.

3. **Improving Digestion**: A well-balanced diet tailored to support your gallbladder can lead to smoother digestion. This means less

discomfort, better nutrient absorption, and an overall improvement in your quality of life.

The Role of Fats in Gallbladder Health

Fats are a critical component of our diet. They provide energy, support cell growth, and aid in the absorption of fat-soluble vitamins (A, D, E, and K). However, when it comes to gallbladder health, not all fats are created equal.

The gallbladder's primary function is to store and release bile, which is essential for digesting fats.

When you consume a meal rich in fats, your gallbladder contracts and releases bile into the small intestine. Bile helps break down fats into smaller droplets, allowing digestive enzymes to do their job more effectively.

However, if you overconsume unhealthy fats or have a predisposition to gallstones, problems can arise. Excessive saturated and trans fats, often found in fried foods, processed snacks, and fatty cuts of meat, can contribute to gallstone formation. These fats prompt the liver to produce more cholesterol, which can lead to the crystallization of cholesterol in the gallbladder.

On the other hand, healthy fats, such as those found in avocados, nuts, seeds, and fatty fish like salmon, can be beneficial for gallbladder health. These fats are more easily digested and less likely to contribute to gallstone formation.

The Low-Fat Approach

Given the gallbladder's role in digesting fats, it's logical that a low-fat diet is often recommended for individuals with gallbladder issues. Here's how a low-fat diet supports gallbladder health:

1. **Reducing Gallstone Formation**: A diet low in saturated and trans fats can help prevent the excessive production of cholesterol in the liver, reducing the risk of gallstones.

2. **Minimizing Gallbladder Contractions**: Lower fat intake means fewer contractions of the gallbladder, which can reduce the likelihood of gallbladder pain and inflammation.

3. **Improving Tolerance**: If you've had gallbladder surgery (cholecystectomy), following a low-fat diet can help manage post-surgery digestive issues. Without a gallbladder to store and release bile, the digestive system can struggle to process large amounts of fat at once.

So, what does a low-fat diet entail? It involves minimizing or eliminating foods high in unhealthy fats, such as:

- Fried foods: French fries, fried chicken, and fried snacks.

- Fatty cuts of meat: Bacon, sausage, and fatty steaks.

- Processed snacks: Chips, crackers, and commercially baked goods.

- Full-fat dairy products: Whole milk, cheese, and butter.

- High-fat sauces and dressings: Cream-based sauces, mayonnaise, and certain salad dressings.

Instead, focus on incorporating healthy fats into your diet, like those found in:

- Avocados: Rich in monounsaturated fats, avocados are a nutritious addition to your meals.
- Nuts and seeds: Almonds, walnuts, chia seeds, and flaxseeds provide healthy fats, fiber, and essential nutrients.
- Fatty fish: Salmon, mackerel, and trout are excellent sources of omega-3 fatty acids.

- Olive oil: Extra virgin olive oil is a staple in Mediterranean diets, known for their heart-healthy benefits.

Embracing High-Fiber Foods

Dietary fiber is another crucial component of a gallbladder-friendly diet. Fiber has numerous health benefits, including promoting regular bowel movements, aiding in weight management, and reducing the risk of heart disease. But how does it relate to gallbladder health?

1. **Reducing Gallstone Risk**: High-fiber diets are associated with a reduced risk of gallstones. Fiber helps regulate cholesterol levels in the bile, preventing the crystallization of cholesterol that can lead to gallstones.

2. **Supporting Digestion**: Fiber-rich foods promote regular bowel movements, preventing constipation. Constipation can lead to gallbladder discomfort and exacerbate existing gallbladder issues.

To incorporate more fiber into your diet, consider adding these foods:

- Whole grains: Choose whole wheat bread, brown rice, quinoa, and oats over refined grains.
- Fruits and vegetables: Aim for a variety of colorful options to maximize your fiber intake.
- Legumes: Beans, lentils, and chickpeas are rich in fiber and protein.
- Nuts and seeds: These not only provide healthy fats but

are also a good source of fiber.

Hydration Matters

While we've discussed the importance of fats and fiber in a gallbladder-friendly diet, let's not forget about hydration. Staying well-hydrated is vital for maintaining gallbladder health and preventing gallstone formation.

Here's why hydration matters:

1. **Diluting Bile**: When you're adequately hydrated, your bile is less concentrated. This reduces the likelihood

of cholesterol crystallizing into gallstones.

2. **Promoting Regular Bowel Movements**: Dehydration can lead to constipation, which can be uncomfortable for individuals with gallbladder issues.

3. **Supporting Overall Health**: Staying hydrated is essential for overall well-being. It helps regulate body temperature, transport nutrients, and eliminate waste products.

To ensure you're drinking enough water, aim for at least eight 8-ounce glasses (about 2 liters) per day. However, individual needs can vary based on factors like climate, activity level, and overall health. Pay attention to your body's signals and drink when you're thirsty.

Chapter Summary

In this chapter, we've explored the foundational principles of a gallbladder diet. We've learned that dietary choices play a crucial role in supporting gallbladder health, preventing gallstone formation, and reducing the risk of complications. By adopting a low-fat diet, incorporating healthy fats, embracing high-fiber foods, and staying adequately hydrated, you can take significant steps toward promoting your gallbladder's well-being and ensuring smoother digestion.

In the upcoming chapters, we'll delve deeper into specific dietary recommendations, meal planning, portion control, and lifestyle factors that can further influence gallbladder health. Armed with this knowledge, you'll be better equipped to make informed choices about your diet and overall health as you navigate the journey towards improved gallbladder function.

CHAPTER 4

Foods to Avoid

Welcome to Chapter 4, where we'll delve into a crucial aspect of a gallbladder-friendly diet: the foods you should avoid. Understanding these dietary no-nos is vital for preventing gallbladder problems, managing existing conditions, and alleviating symptoms. Let's explore the foods that can exacerbate gallbladder issues and learn how to make healthier choices.

The Culprits: Foods that Aggravate Gallbladder Problems

Certain foods can be particularly troublesome for your gallbladder. They can trigger painful symptoms, contribute to gallstone formation, or worsen existing conditions. Let's identify these dietary culprits:

1. **Fatty Foods**: High-fat foods are at the top of the list of gallbladder antagonists. They stimulate the gallbladder to release bile, which can be problematic if

you have gallstones or a compromised gallbladder.

- *Avoid:* Fried foods (French fries, fried chicken), fatty cuts of meat (bacon, sausage), full-fat dairy (whole milk, cheese), high-fat sauces and dressings.

2. **Processed Foods**: Many processed foods are laden with unhealthy fats, additives, and preservatives. They offer little nutritional value and can exacerbate gallbladder problems.

- *Avoid:* Packaged snacks (chips,

crackers), fast food, frozen meals, and commercially baked goods.

3. **Spicy Foods**: Spicy foods can irritate the digestive tract and trigger discomfort, particularly if you have a sensitive gallbladder.

   - *Moderate:* If you enjoy spicy foods, consume them in moderation and pay attention to how your body reacts.

4. **High-Cholesterol Foods**: Diets high in cholesterol can contribute to the formation of cholesterol-based

gallstones, a common gallbladder issue.

- *Avoid:* Organ meats (liver, kidney), egg yolks, and excessive consumption of high-cholesterol animal products.

5. **Rapid Weight Loss Diets**: Crash diets or very low-calorie diets that lead to rapid weight loss can increase the risk of gallstones.

- *Avoid:* Extreme calorie restriction or unbalanced diets

lacking essential nutrients.

6. **Sugary Foods and Beverages**: Excessive sugar intake can lead to weight gain and obesity, which are risk factors for gallstone formation.

   o *Moderate:* Limit sugary snacks, sugary drinks, and excessive consumption of sweets.

7. **Heavy, Creamy Sauces**: Cream-based sauces are high in fat and can be hard to digest, especially if you have gallbladder issues.

- *Avoid:* Alfredo sauce, creamy soups, and rich gravies.

8. **Caffeine and Carbonated Beverages**: Caffeine can stimulate the gallbladder to contract, potentially causing discomfort.

   - *Moderate:* Limit caffeine intake from coffee, tea, and energy drinks. Carbonated beverages can also cause bloating and discomfort in some individuals.

Reading Food Labels

One of the essential skills in adopting a gallbladder-friendly diet is learning to read food labels. Manufacturers are required to list the ingredients and nutritional information on packaged foods, helping you make informed choices. Here's what to look for:

1. **Total Fat**: Pay attention to the total fat content per serving. Aim for foods with lower fat content, especially saturated and trans fats.

2. **Saturated Fat**: This type of fat is found in animal products and some processed foods. It's best to

keep saturated fat intake to a minimum.

3. **Trans Fat**: Avoid products that contain trans fats altogether. They are often found in partially hydrogenated oils and have been linked to various health issues.

4. **Cholesterol**: If you're at risk of gallstones, keep an eye on the cholesterol content in foods. High-cholesterol foods can contribute to gallstone formation.

5. **Fiber**: Foods high in fiber can help promote

gallbladder health. Look for products with higher fiber content.

6. **Sugar**: Limit foods and beverages with added sugars. These can contribute to weight gain, which is a risk factor for gallstones.

7. **Ingredients**: Read the list of ingredients. Be wary of processed foods with long lists of additives and preservatives.

The Importance of Portion Control

While some foods are best avoided altogether, portion control plays a vital role in managing gallbladder health. Here's why it matters:

1. **Preventing Overloading**: Eating large, heavy meals can overwhelm your gallbladder, especially if you have gallstones or a compromised gallbladder.

2. **Balancing Fat Intake**: Even when consuming healthier fats, such as those found in avocados or nuts, portion control is crucial. These fats are nutritious but calorie-dense.

3. **Avoiding Overeating**: Overeating, in general, can

lead to discomfort, indigestion, and potentially trigger gallbladder symptoms.

Meal Planning with Gallbladder Health in Mind

Effective meal planning is a cornerstone of a gallbladder-friendly diet. Here are some practical tips:

1. **Balanced Meals**: Aim for balanced meals that include lean proteins, whole grains, plenty of vegetables, and healthy fats in appropriate portions.

2. **Frequent, Smaller Meals**: Consider eating smaller, more frequent meals throughout the day. This can prevent overloading your gallbladder.

3. **Healthy Cooking Methods**: Choose healthier cooking methods like baking, grilling, steaming, or sautéing instead of frying.

4. **High-Fiber Choices**: Opt for high-fiber foods like whole grains, legumes, fruits, and vegetables to promote digestive regularity.

5. **Hydration**: Stay well-hydrated by drinking plenty of water throughout the day.

6. **Mindful Eating**: Pay attention to your body's signals of hunger and fullness. Eating mindfully can help prevent overeating.

7. **Consult a Dietitian**: If you're unsure how to create gallbladder-friendly meal plans, consider consulting a registered dietitian. They can provide personalized guidance.

Chapter Summary

In Chapter 4, we've explored the foods that can exacerbate gallbladder problems and learned about the importance of portion control and reading food labels. By avoiding or moderating certain foods and making informed choices, you can support your gallbladder's health, reduce the risk of gallstone formation, and alleviate symptoms. In the next chapter, we'll shift our focus to the positive side of dietary choices by exploring gallbladder-friendly foods that can promote digestive well-being and overall health.

CHAPTER 5

Foods to Embrace - Promoting Gallbladder Health

Welcome to Chapter 5, where we shift our focus from the foods to avoid to the foods you should embrace for promoting gallbladder health. These gallbladder-friendly foods are your allies in preventing gallstones, managing gallbladder issues, and supporting overall digestive well-being. Let's explore the nutrient-rich options that can make a positive difference in your diet.

1. Fiber-Rich Foods

Fiber is a superstar when it comes to gallbladder health. It helps regulate cholesterol levels in the bile, preventing the formation of cholesterol-based gallstones. Additionally, fiber promotes regular bowel movements, reducing the risk of constipation, which can exacerbate gallbladder discomfort. Here are some fiber-rich foods to incorporate into your diet:

- **Whole Grains**: Opt for whole grains like brown rice, whole wheat pasta, quinoa, and oats. These grains are not only rich in fiber but also provide essential nutrients.

- **Fruits and Vegetables**: A colorful array of fruits and vegetables is your ticket to fiber-rich goodness. Berries, apples, pears, broccoli, carrots, and leafy greens are excellent choices.

- **Legumes**: Beans, lentils, and chickpeas are not only high in fiber but also pack a protein punch, making them an excellent addition to your meals.

- **Nuts and Seeds**: Almonds, chia seeds, flaxseeds, and walnuts are not only a source of healthy fats but also provide fiber and a variety of nutrients.

2. Lean Proteins

Protein is essential for overall health, and choosing lean sources can support your gallbladder. Lean proteins are less likely to trigger gallbladder contractions and discomfort, making them a valuable addition to your diet. Here are some options:

- **Poultry**: Skinless chicken and turkey are excellent sources of lean protein.

Remove the skin to minimize saturated fat content.

- **Fish**: Fatty fish like salmon, mackerel, and trout provide healthy omega-3 fatty acids along with protein. These fats are beneficial for gallbladder health.

- **Plant-Based Proteins**: If you're following a vegetarian or vegan diet, consider tofu, tempeh, and legumes as sources of protein.

3. Healthy Fats

While it's essential to limit unhealthy fats, your body still needs healthy fats to function correctly. These fats are less likely to trigger gallbladder contractions and can even support gallbladder health. Incorporate these sources of healthy fats into your meals:

- **Avocados**: Avocados are rich in monounsaturated fats, which are good for your heart and gallbladder. Use them in salads, sandwiches, or as a spread.
- **Nuts and Seeds**: Almonds, walnuts, chia seeds, and flaxseeds are not only fiber-rich but also provide healthy fats.

- **Fatty Fish**: Salmon, mackerel, and trout are rich in omega-3 fatty acids, which have anti-inflammatory properties and can support gallbladder health.

- **Olive Oil**: Extra virgin olive oil is a staple in Mediterranean diets and offers numerous health benefits, including support for gallbladder health.

4. Low-Fat Dairy

Dairy products can be a source of calcium and protein, but they can also be high in saturated fats. Opt for low-fat or fat-free dairy options to reap the benefits without overloading your gallbladder. Here are some choices:

- **Low-Fat or Fat-Free Milk**: These options provide calcium and vitamin D without the saturated fat found in whole milk.
- **Greek Yogurt**: Greek yogurt is higher in protein and lower in fat compared to regular yogurt.
- **Low-Fat Cheese**: Some types of cheese are available in low-fat varieties. These

can be used in moderation to add flavor to your meals.

5. Fruits and Vegetables

Fruits and vegetables are rich in vitamins, minerals, antioxidants, and dietary fiber, all of which contribute to overall health and support gallbladder function. Here's how you can make the most of these nutritional powerhouses:

- **Variety**: Aim to eat a wide variety of fruits and vegetables to ensure you receive a broad spectrum of nutrients.

- **Fresh and Frozen**: Fresh and frozen produce are both excellent choices. Choose what's in season for the best flavor and nutrition.
- **Cooking Methods**: Steaming, roasting, and grilling are healthy ways to prepare vegetables while preserving their nutrient content.

6. Water-Rich Foods

Staying hydrated is crucial for gallbladder health, as it helps prevent the bile from becoming overly concentrated. Some foods have a high water content and can contribute to your daily hydration needs:

- **Cucumbers**: Cucumbers are over 95% water and can be a refreshing addition to salads and sandwiches.

- **Watermelon**: Watermelon is not only delicious but also a great source of hydration, especially on hot days.

- **Oranges**: Citrus fruits like oranges are not only hydrating but also provide essential vitamins and minerals.

- **Leafy Greens**: Lettuce, spinach, and other leafy

greens have a high water content, making them excellent choices for salads.

7. Herbal Teas

Herbal teas can be soothing for the digestive system and may help alleviate gallbladder discomfort. Some herbal teas are known for their potential benefits:

- **Peppermint Tea**: Peppermint tea may help relax the muscles in the digestive tract and relieve symptoms like bloating and gas.

- **Ginger Tea**: Ginger has anti-inflammatory properties and may aid in digestion. It's also known for its soothing effect on the stomach.

8. Whole, Unprocessed Foods

Choosing whole, unprocessed foods whenever possible is a cornerstone of a gallbladder-friendly diet. Processed foods often contain unhealthy fats, additives, and preservatives that can exacerbate gallbladder problems. Whole foods, on the other hand, are naturally nutrient-rich and support overall health.

9. Moderation with Spices and Seasonings

While spicy foods can irritate the digestive tract and trigger discomfort in some individuals, moderate use of spices and seasonings can add flavor to your meals without causing issues. Experiment with spices like turmeric, cumin, and coriander, which have anti-inflammatory properties.

10. Mindful Eating

Last but not least, practicing mindful eating is essential for gallbladder health. Pay attention to your body's signals of hunger and fullness, and eat at a relaxed pace. Overeating can lead to discomfort and indigestion, potentially triggering gallbladder symptoms.

Chapter Summary

In Chapter 5, we've explored the foods you should embrace to promote gallbladder health. These nutrient-rich options include fiber-rich foods, lean proteins, healthy fats, low-fat dairy, fruits, vegetables, water-rich foods, herbal teas, whole unprocessed foods, and mindful eating practices. By incorporating these gallbladder-friendly foods into your diet and making informed choices, you can support your gallbladder, reduce the risk of gallstone formation, and enjoy improved digestive well-being. In the next chapter, we'll put this knowledge into action by providing sample meal plans and practical tips for planning gallbladder-friendly meals.

CHAPTER 6

Practical Meal Planning for Gallbladder Health

In Chapter 6, we take the knowledge gained from the previous chapters and put it into action by providing practical meal planning guidance for promoting gallbladder health. Meal planning is essential for ensuring that your dietary choices align with the principles of a gallbladder-friendly diet. We'll explore sample meal plans and offer practical tips for creating balanced, delicious, and nutritious meals that support your gallbladder and overall well-being.

Sample Meal Plans

Let's dive into some sample meal plans that incorporate gallbladder-friendly foods and dietary principles. Remember that these plans are just examples, and you can customize them to suit your taste preferences and dietary needs.

Meal Plan 1: A Balanced Breakfast

Breakfast: Oatmeal with Fresh Berries and Almonds

- Start your day with a bowl of oatmeal made with water or low-fat milk.

- Top it with fresh berries (such as blueberries or strawberries) for added fiber and antioxidants.

- Sprinkle a handful of almonds or chopped nuts for healthy fats and protein.

Snack: Greek Yogurt with Honey and Banana

- Enjoy a small serving of Greek yogurt, which is high in protein and low in fat.

- Drizzle honey for sweetness and add banana slices for

additional nutrients and fiber.

Lunch: Grilled Chicken Salad

- Prepare a salad with leafy greens (like spinach or kale) and colorful vegetables (tomatoes, cucumbers, and bell peppers).
- Add grilled chicken breast for lean protein.
- Dress with a vinaigrette made from olive oil, lemon juice, and herbs.

Snack: Carrot Sticks with Hummus

- Carrot sticks are a crunchy, low-calorie snack.
- Pair them with hummus for extra flavor and protein.

Dinner: Baked Salmon with Quinoa and Steamed Broccoli

- Bake a salmon fillet seasoned with herbs and a drizzle of olive oil.
- Serve it alongside cooked quinoa, a whole grain high in fiber.
- Complete the meal with steamed broccoli for added vitamins and fiber.

Snack (Optional): A Small Portion of Fresh Fruit

- If you need a late-night snack, opt for a small portion of fresh fruit, such as an apple or pear.

Meal Plan 2: A Vegetarian Day

Breakfast: Avocado Toast with Poached Egg

- Spread mashed avocado on whole wheat toast.
- Top it with a poached egg for protein and extra flavor.
- Sprinkle with a pinch of black pepper.

Snack: Almonds and Dried Cranberries

- A handful of almonds and dried cranberries provide a mix of healthy fats, fiber, and a touch of sweetness.

Lunch: Quinoa and Chickpea Salad

- Combine cooked quinoa, canned chickpeas, diced cucumbers, cherry tomatoes, and fresh parsley.
- Drizzle with a lemon and olive oil dressing.

Snack: Sliced Cucumber with Greek Yogurt Dip

- Slice cucumber into sticks and enjoy with a side of Greek yogurt mixed with dill and lemon juice for a refreshing snack.

Dinner: Stir-Fried Tofu with Mixed Vegetables and Brown Rice

- Stir-fry tofu cubes with a variety of colorful vegetables like bell peppers, broccoli, and carrots.
- Season with a low-sodium soy sauce or teriyaki sauce.
- Serve over cooked brown rice for a wholesome meal.

Snack (Optional): Sliced Bell Peppers with Hummus

- Bell pepper strips are a crunchy and low-calorie option for dipping in hummus.

Meal Planning Tips for Gallbladder Health

Now that we've explored some sample meal plans, let's delve into practical tips for meal planning that align with gallbladder health principles:

1. Balance Macronutrients

Aim to include a balance of carbohydrates, proteins, and healthy fats in each meal. This balance helps stabilize blood sugar levels and supports overall digestive well-being.

2. Choose Lean Proteins

Opt for lean protein sources like chicken, turkey, fish, tofu, and legumes. These options are less likely to trigger gallbladder contractions.

3. Go for Whole Grains

Choose whole grains like brown rice, quinoa, whole wheat pasta, and oats over refined grains.

Whole grains are higher in fiber, which is beneficial for gallbladder health.

4. Incorporate Fiber-Rich Foods

Fruits, vegetables, legumes, nuts, and seeds are excellent sources of dietary fiber. Aim to include these in your meals to support digestive regularity.

5. Mind Your Portions

Practice portion control to prevent overloading your digestive system and gallbladder. Eating smaller, more frequent meals can be helpful.

6. Stay Hydrated

Drink plenty of water throughout the day to keep your bile from becoming too concentrated. Herbal teas and water-rich foods like fruits and vegetables can contribute to your hydration needs.

7. Embrace Healthy Fats

Incorporate healthy fats like avocados, nuts, seeds, and olive oil into your diet, but do so in moderation. These fats are nutritious but calorie-dense.

8. Minimize Processed Foods

Limit processed foods, which often contain unhealthy fats, additives, and preservatives that can aggravate gallbladder issues.

9. Experiment with Herbs and Spices

Herbs and spices like ginger, turmeric, and peppermint can have digestive benefits. Experiment with them in your cooking to add flavor and potential health benefits.

10. Plan Ahead

Consider planning your meals for the week in advance. This can help you make healthier choices and avoid last-minute, less nutritious options.

11. Listen to Your Body

Pay attention to your body's signals of hunger and fullness. Eating mindfully can prevent overeating and discomfort.

12. Consult a Dietitian

If you're unsure how to create gallbladder-friendly meal plans or have specific dietary concerns, consider consulting a registered dietitian. They can provide personalized guidance based on your needs and preferences.

Conclusion

In Chapter 6, we've explored practical meal planning for gallbladder health, providing sample meal plans and essential tips to create balanced, delicious, and nutritious meals that support your gallbladder and overall well-being. By incorporating these principles into your daily eating habits, you can take proactive steps towards promoting gallbladder health, reducing the risk of gallstone formation, and enjoying improved digestive comfort. In the next chapter, we'll discuss lifestyle factors and habits

that complement your dietary
choices for a holistic approach to
gallbladder well-being.

CHAPTER 7

Lifestyle Factors for Gallbladder Health

Welcome to Chapter 7, where we delve into the lifestyle factors and habits that complement your dietary choices for a holistic approach to gallbladder health. While a gallbladder-friendly diet is crucial, other aspects of your lifestyle also play a significant role in supporting your gallbladder's well-being. Let's explore how factors such as physical activity, stress management, and sleep contribute to a healthier gallbladder and overall digestive comfort.

1. Stay Physically Active

Regular physical activity is not only beneficial for maintaining a healthy weight but also for promoting gallbladder health. Exercise helps stimulate digestion, supports healthy metabolism, and may reduce the risk of gallstone formation. Here's how to incorporate physical activity into your routine:

- **Aim for Regularity**: Aim for at least 150 minutes of

moderate-intensity aerobic activity per week, such as brisk walking, cycling, or swimming.

- **Strength Training**: Incorporate strength training exercises at least two days a week. Building muscle mass can boost metabolism and support overall health.

- **Stay Active Throughout the Day**: In addition to dedicated workouts, find ways to stay active throughout the day. Take short walks, use the stairs, and stand up and stretch periodically.

2. Manage Stress

Stress can have a significant impact on your digestive system, including your gallbladder. Chronic stress can lead to imbalances in the digestive process and may exacerbate gallbladder symptoms. Here's how to manage stress effectively:

- **Practice Relaxation Techniques**: Engage in relaxation techniques such as deep breathing, meditation, and mindfulness. These practices can help calm the mind and reduce stress.

- **Stay Active**: Physical activity is not only good for your body but also for your mental well-being. Exercise releases endorphins, which are natural mood enhancers.

- **Prioritize Self-Care**: Dedicate time to activities that bring you joy and relaxation. Whether it's reading, spending time with loved ones, or enjoying a hobby, self-care is essential for managing stress.

3. Prioritize Sleep

Quality sleep is crucial for overall health, including gallbladder health. Poor sleep patterns can disrupt digestion and lead to various health issues, including weight gain. Here's how to improve your sleep:

- **Establish a Routine**: Go to bed and wake up at the same time every day, even on weekends. A consistent sleep schedule helps regulate your body's internal clock.
- **Create a Relaxing Bedtime Ritual**: Engage in calming activities before

bed, such as reading, taking a warm bath, or practicing gentle stretches.

- **Create a Comfortable Sleep Environment**: Ensure your sleep environment is conducive to rest. Use blackout curtains, maintain a comfortable room temperature, and invest in a comfortable mattress and pillows.

4. Avoid Rapid Weight Fluctuations

Extreme weight loss or gain can affect gallbladder function and increase the risk of gallstone formation. Avoid crash diets or sudden changes in eating habits that lead to rapid weight fluctuations.

- **Focus on Sustainable Changes**: Instead of aiming for quick fixes, focus on making sustainable changes to your diet and lifestyle that support long-term health.

5. Stay Hydrated

We've already discussed the importance of hydration for gallbladder health. Drinking plenty of water helps prevent the bile from becoming too concentrated and reduces the risk of gallstone formation.

- **Carry a Water Bottle**: Keep a reusable water bottle with you throughout the day to remind yourself to stay hydrated.

- **Set Hydration Goals**: Aim to drink a certain amount of water by specific times of the day to track your hydration progress.

6. Limit Alcohol Consumption

Excessive alcohol consumption can disrupt digestive processes and contribute to gallbladder discomfort. If you choose to drink alcohol, do so in moderation.

- **Moderation is Key**: For those who choose to consume alcohol, moderation means up to one drink per day for women and up to two drinks per day for men.

7. Avoid Smoking

Smoking is associated with various health issues, including gallbladder problems. It can increase the risk of gallstone formation and worsen gallbladder symptoms.

- **Seek Support to Quit**: If you smoke, consider seeking support to quit. Quitting smoking has numerous benefits for your overall health.

8. Listen to Your Body

Ultimately, one of the most important lifestyle factors for gallbladder health is listening to your body. Pay attention to how different foods, activities, and situations affect your digestion and well-being.

- **Keep a Food and Symptom Journal**: Consider keeping a journal to track your dietary choices and any symptoms you experience. This can help you identify patterns and make informed decisions.

- **Trust Your Intuition**: If a certain food or activity doesn't feel right for your body, trust your intuition and make choices that support your well-being.

Conclusion

Chapter 7 underscores the importance of lifestyle factors and habits that complement your dietary choices for promoting gallbladder health. Staying physically active, managing stress, prioritizing sleep, avoiding rapid weight fluctuations, staying hydrated, limiting alcohol consumption, avoiding smoking, and listening to your body are all essential components of a holistic approach to gallbladder well-being. By integrating these practices into your daily life, you can further support your gallbladder's health, reduce the risk of gallstone formation, and enjoy improved digestive comfort. In the final chapter, we'll summarize the key takeaways from our exploration of gallbladder health and offer some closing thoughts on your journey towards better digestive well-being.

CHAPTER 8

Conclusion - Your Journey to Gallbladder Health

Congratulations on completing this journey through the intricacies of gallbladder health! In this final chapter, we'll summarize the key takeaways from our exploration of gallbladder health and offer some closing thoughts to guide you on your path towards better digestive well-being.

Key Takeaways

Let's recap the essential lessons we've covered in this book:

Chapter 1: Understanding the Gallbladder

- We began by introducing you to the gallbladder, an often-overlooked organ that plays a crucial role in digestion by storing and releasing bile.

Chapter 2: Gallbladder Conditions and Symptoms

- In Chapter 2, we explored common gallbladder conditions like gallstones and gallbladder inflammation, and we discussed the symptoms associated with these conditions.

Chapter 3: Risk Factors and Prevention

- We highlighted the risk factors for gallbladder problems and discussed preventive measures, including maintaining a healthy weight and avoiding rapid weight loss.

Chapter 4: Foods to Avoid

- Chapter 4 delved into the foods you should avoid, as

certain dietary choices can exacerbate gallbladder issues. We emphasized the importance of avoiding fatty, processed, spicy, and high-cholesterol foods.

Chapter 5: Foods to Embrace

- In Chapter 5, we explored the foods you should embrace for promoting gallbladder health. Fiber-rich foods, lean proteins, healthy fats, and whole, unprocessed foods were highlighted as allies in your journey to digestive well-being.

Chapter 6: Practical Meal Planning

- Chapter 6 provided practical meal planning guidance with sample meal plans and tips for creating balanced, nutritious, and delicious meals that support your gallbladder.

Chapter 7: Lifestyle Factors for Gallbladder Health

- We discussed lifestyle factors in Chapter 7, including the importance of staying physically active, managing stress, prioritizing sleep, avoiding rapid weight fluctuations, staying hydrated, limiting alcohol consumption, avoiding smoking, and listening to your body.

Closing Thoughts

As you reflect on your journey to gallbladder health, here are some closing thoughts to guide you on your path:

1. Knowledge Empowers

Understanding your gallbladder and the factors that influence its health is empowering. Armed with knowledge, you can make informed choices about your diet, lifestyle, and overall well-being.

2. Balance is Key

Maintaining a balanced approach to gallbladder health is crucial. Strive for moderation in your dietary choices, portion sizes, physical activity, and stress management. Balance ensures that you address the needs of your body while minimizing the risk of gallbladder issues.

3. Customization Matters

Your journey to gallbladder health is personal. What works for one person may not work for another.

It's essential to customize your approach based on your unique needs, preferences, and any existing gallbladder conditions.

4. Progress Over Perfection

Remember that achieving gallbladder health is about progress, not perfection. Don't be too hard on yourself if you occasionally indulge in a less healthy meal or experience setbacks. What matters is your overall commitment to supporting your gallbladder's well-being.

5. Seek Professional Guidance

If you have existing gallbladder conditions or specific dietary concerns, consider seeking professional guidance. A registered dietitian or healthcare provider can provide personalized recommendations tailored to your situation.

6. Listen to Your Body

Your body often provides signals and cues about what it needs. Pay attention to how different foods, activities, and situations affect your digestion and well-being. Trust your intuition and make choices that support your health.

7. Long-Term Health

Gallbladder health is not just about managing symptoms; it's about promoting long-term well-being. By adopting a holistic approach that considers diet, lifestyle, and overall health, you can enjoy improved digestive comfort and enhanced quality of life.

Closing Remarks

Your journey to gallbladder health is a testament to your commitment to well-being. By understanding the importance of your gallbladder, making informed dietary choices, embracing a balanced lifestyle, and prioritizing self-care, you've taken significant steps towards supporting your digestive comfort.

It's important to remember that achieving and maintaining gallbladder health is an ongoing process. As you move forward, continue to explore new recipes, discover physical activities you enjoy, and refine your stress management techniques. Be patient with yourself and celebrate your successes, no matter how small they may seem.

Lastly, your journey towards gallbladder health can have a positive ripple effect on your overall well-being. By nurturing your digestive system, you're contributing to your overall health and vitality. Your body will thank you for the care and attention you've given it.

Thank you for joining us on this journey through gallbladder health. We hope this book has provided you with valuable insights and practical guidance to support your path towards a healthier, more comfortable digestive life. As you continue your journey, may your gallbladder be a source of well-being and vitality, allowing you to savor life's many flavors with joy and ease.

CHAPTER 9

Frequently Asked Questions About Gallbladder Health

In this final chapter, we address some common questions and concerns that readers may have about gallbladder health. Whether you've recently been diagnosed with a gallbladder condition, are seeking preventive measures, or simply want to better understand this crucial organ, this chapter provides answers to frequently asked questions to further enhance your knowledge.

1. What Does the Gallbladder Do?

The gallbladder is a small, pear-shaped organ located beneath the liver. Its primary function is to store bile, a digestive fluid produced by the liver. When you eat, especially when consuming fatty foods, the gallbladder contracts and releases bile into the small intestine. Bile helps break down dietary fats, making them easier to digest and absorb.

2. What Are Common Gallbladder Conditions?

Two of the most common gallbladder conditions are:

- **Gallstones**: These are solid particles that form in the gallbladder. They can be made of cholesterol, bilirubin, or a combination of both. Gallstones can cause pain and discomfort if they block the bile ducts.

- **Cholecystitis**: This is inflammation of the gallbladder, often caused by gallstones. It can lead to severe pain, fever, and infection.

3. What Are the Symptoms of Gallbladder Problems?

Gallbladder problems can manifest with various symptoms, including:

- **Abdominal pain**: Typically felt in the upper right or center of the abdomen, this pain can be severe and may radiate to the back or right shoulder blade.

- **Nausea and vomiting**: Nausea and vomiting may accompany gallbladder attacks.

- **Indigestion**: You might experience bloating, gas, and

a feeling of fullness after meals.

- **Fever and chills**: These symptoms can be a sign of gallbladder inflammation (cholecystitis).

4. Can Diet Prevent Gallbladder Problems?

A healthy diet can play a significant role in preventing gallbladder problems, especially gallstones. Key dietary principles include:

- **Balanced Eating**: Consume a balanced diet that includes a variety of fruits, vegetables, lean proteins, and whole grains.

- **Fiber-Rich Foods**: Foods high in fiber, such as whole grains, fruits, and vegetables, may help prevent gallstone formation.

- **Healthy Fats**: Incorporate healthy fats like those found in avocados, nuts, and olive oil into your diet.

- **Moderation**: Limit your intake of high-fat, processed, and spicy foods.

- **Stay Hydrated**: Drinking plenty of water can help prevent the bile from becoming too concentrated.

5. Are There Specific Foods That Can Help My Gallbladder?

While there are no "magic" foods that guarantee gallbladder health, some dietary choices can be beneficial. These include:

- **Fiber-rich foods**: Fruits, vegetables, and whole grains can help regulate cholesterol levels in the bile and promote digestive regularity.

- **Lean proteins**: Choose lean sources of protein like chicken, turkey, fish, and tofu to minimize gallbladder contractions.

- **Healthy fats**: Incorporate healthy fats from sources like avocados, nuts, seeds, and olive oil into your meals.

6. Can I Still Enjoy Flavors and Spices on a Gallbladder-Friendly Diet?

Absolutely! A gallbladder-friendly diet doesn't mean sacrificing flavor. You can use herbs and spices to add taste to your meals without triggering discomfort. Many herbs and spices, such as ginger, turmeric, and cumin, may even have digestive benefits.

7. How Can I Manage Gallbladder Pain at Home?

If you're experiencing gallbladder pain at home, you can try the following:

- **Rest**: Lie down and try to relax. Sometimes, resting can alleviate mild pain.

- **Heat**: Applying a warm compress or heating pad to the area may provide relief.

- **Over-the-Counter Pain Medication**: Non-prescription pain relievers like ibuprofen or acetaminophen may help manage mild pain. However, consult a healthcare provider before taking any medication.

8. When Should I Seek Medical Attention for Gallbladder Pain?

It's essential to seek medical attention if you experience severe or persistent gallbladder pain, especially if it's accompanied by fever, chills, or jaundice (yellowing of the skin or eyes). These symptoms can indicate a more serious condition that requires medical evaluation and treatment.

9. What Are the Treatment Options for Gallbladder Problems?

The treatment for gallbladder problems depends on the specific condition:

- **Gallstones**: Treatment options include medications to dissolve stones, minimally invasive procedures to remove them, or surgical removal of the gallbladder (cholecystectomy).
- **Cholecystitis**: Treatment may involve hospitalization, fasting to rest the gallbladder, antibiotics, and

potentially surgery to remove the gallbladder.

Your healthcare provider will recommend the most appropriate treatment based on your diagnosis and individual circumstances.

10. Can I Live Normally Without a Gallbladder?

Yes, you can live a normal, healthy life without a gallbladder. The gallbladder is not a vital organ, and your body can adapt to its absence. After gallbladder removal surgery (cholecystectomy), you may need to make some dietary adjustments to accommodate the absence of the organ, but most people can resume their regular activities.

11. Are There Any Long-Term Dietary Considerations After Gallbladder Removal?

After gallbladder removal, some individuals may experience changes in digestion, such as increased frequency of bowel movements or loose stools, especially after consuming high-fat meals. To manage these changes, it may be helpful to:

- **Gradually Introduce Fats**: Gradually reintroduce

fats into your diet and pay attention to how your body responds.

- **Smaller, More Frequent Meals**: Eating smaller, more frequent meals can help prevent digestive discomfort.
- **Monitor Trigger Foods**: Identify any specific foods that tend to trigger digestive symptoms and consider reducing or avoiding them.

12. Can Gallbladder Problems Reoccur After Surgery?

In some cases, gallbladder problems can reoccur even after gallbladder removal surgery.

However, this is relatively rare. It's essential to follow your healthcare provider's post-surgery recommendations and maintain a healthy lifestyle to reduce the risk of future issues.

13. Can Lifestyle Changes Prevent Gallbladder Problems If I Have a Family History?

While family history can influence your risk of gallbladder problems, adopting a healthy lifestyle can still be beneficial in reducing that risk. Maintaining a healthy weight, eating a balanced diet, staying physically active, and managing stress are all valuable preventive measures.

14. What If I Have Other Digestive Issues Alongside Gallbladder Problems?

If you have other digestive issues, such as irritable bowel syndrome (IBS) or gastroesophageal reflux disease (GERD), it's essential to work closely with a healthcare provider or gastroenterologist to manage these conditions in conjunction with your gallbladder concerns. Comprehensive care can address the full spectrum of digestive health.

Conclusion

In this final chapter, we've addressed common questions and concerns about gallbladder health, providing you with valuable insights to enhance your understanding of this essential organ. Whether you're seeking preventive measures or managing gallbladder issues, knowledge is a powerful tool in promoting digestive well-being.

As you continue your journey towards gallbladder health, remember that you have the ability to make informed choices about your diet, lifestyle, and overall well-being. Whether you're striving to prevent gallbladder problems or navigating life after gallbladder removal, your commitment to digestive comfort and long-term health is commendable.

If you have specific concerns or require personalized guidance, don't hesitate to consult with a healthcare provider or registered dietitian. They can offer tailored recommendations to support your individual needs and help you achieve the best possible digestive health.

Thank you for joining us on this exploration of gallbladder health. We hope this book has provided you with valuable information and answers to your questions, empowering you to make choices that enhance your digestive well-being. May your journey be marked by comfort, vitality, and a deeper understanding of your body's unique needs.

CHAPTER 10

Resources and Additional Information

In this final chapter, we provide a valuable resource guide and additional information to support your ongoing journey towards gallbladder health. Whether you're looking for reputable organizations, trusted websites, helpful books, or practical tools, this chapter aims to connect you with the resources you need to continue your pursuit of digestive well-being.

1. Reputable Organizations

- **American College of Gastroenterology (ACG)**: The ACG is a trusted source for information on gastrointestinal health, including gallbladder conditions and digestive disorders. Their website offers patient education materials and resources.

- **The American Gastroenterological Association (AGA)**: The AGA provides resources related to digestive health and disorders. They offer a wide range of information for patients and healthcare professionals.

- **National Institute of Diabetes and Digestive and Kidney Diseases (NIDDK)**: NIDDK, part of the National Institutes of Health (NIH), conducts research and provides resources on various digestive diseases, including gallstones and gallbladder problems.

2. Reliable Websites

- **Mayo Clinic**: Mayo Clinic's website provides

comprehensive, easy-to-understand information on gallbladder health, including symptoms, causes, and treatment options.

- **MedlinePlus**: A service of the National Library of Medicine, MedlinePlus offers reliable information on gallbladder conditions, prevention, and treatment.

- **WebMD**: WebMD's digestive health section covers a wide range of topics related to the gallbladder, including diet, symptoms, and medical procedures.

3. Helpful Books

- **"The Complete Idiot's Guide to the Gallbladder" by Deborah W. Bine**: This book offers a user-friendly guide to understanding gallbladder health, including explanations of common conditions and dietary recommendations.

- **"Eating for Gastroparesis: Guidelines, Tips & Recipes" by Crystal Zaborowski Saltrelli**: While not specific to gallbladder health, this book provides valuable insights into managing digestive issues through diet.

- **"The Digestive Health Solution" by Benjamin Brown**: This book explores the connection between digestive health and overall well-being, offering practical advice on diet, lifestyle, and gut health.

4. Mobile Apps

- **MyFitnessPal**: This popular app can help you track your food intake, monitor your macronutrient ratios, and set dietary goals to support gallbladder health.

- **Calm**: Managing stress is essential for digestive well-being. Calm is a meditation and relaxation app that can help you reduce stress and anxiety.

- **MyPlate by Livestrong**: MyPlate is a nutrition and calorie tracking app that can assist you in making healthy dietary choices to support your gallbladder.

5. Support Groups

- **Gallbladder Disease and Gallbladder Removal Support Group (Facebook)**: Online support groups, like this one on Facebook, provide a platform to connect with others who have experienced gallbladder problems, share advice, and find emotional support.

6. Recipe Websites

- **EatingWell**: EatingWell offers a collection of gallbladder-friendly recipes that focus on whole, nutritious ingredients.

- **Allrecipes**: This website features a variety of recipes, including options for those with dietary restrictions or preferences related to gallbladder health.

7. Healthcare Providers

- **Gastroenterologist**: A gastroenterologist is a medical specialist with expertise in diagnosing and treating digestive disorders, including gallbladder conditions. If you have specific concerns or symptoms, consider scheduling an appointment with a gastroenterologist for evaluation and guidance.

- **Registered Dietitian**: A registered dietitian can provide personalized dietary recommendations tailored to your gallbladder health needs. They can help you create a meal plan that aligns with your goals and preferences.

8. Educational Materials

- **Printable Food Journal**: Keeping a food journal can help you track your dietary choices and identify patterns that may affect your gallbladder health. Many templates are available online that you can print and use.

- **Gallbladder Diet Guidelines**: Some websites and healthcare organizations offer printable gallbladder diet guidelines that you can reference and use as a dietary resource.

9. Dietary Apps

- **Low-FODMAP Diet Apps**: If you have digestive conditions in addition to gallbladder issues, apps like "Monash University Low

FODMAP Diet" can be useful for managing your diet.

10. Online Gallbladder Forums

- **Patient.info Forums**: Online forums like those on Patient.info allow individuals to share their experiences with gallbladder conditions, exchange advice, and offer support to one another.

11. Health Insurance Information

- If you have health insurance, your provider may offer

resources and tools to help you navigate your healthcare needs, including consultations with specialists.

12. Local Support Groups

- Investigate whether there are local support groups or health organizations in your area that focus on digestive health. They may provide in-person support and educational events.

Conclusion

Chapter 10 serves as a valuable resource guide and source of additional information to support your ongoing journey towards gallbladder health. Whether you're seeking reputable organizations, trusted websites, helpful books, practical tools, or connections with others who share your experiences, these resources can be instrumental in helping you make informed choices and enhance your digestive well-being.

Remember that every person's journey to gallbladder health is unique. You may find certain resources more beneficial than others, and it's essential to tailor your approach to your specific needs and circumstances. Whether you're looking for dietary guidance, medical information, emotional support, or practical tools, the resources provided in this chapter can assist you in making informed decisions and taking proactive steps towards better digestive comfort and overall well-being.

As you continue your journey, may these resources serve as valuable companions, empowering you to navigate the complexities of gallbladder health with confidence and resilience. Your commitment to digestive well-being is

commendable, and we wish you
continued success in your pursuit
of a healthy and comfortable life.

9 798886 956282 1